HOW TO
MANAGE DIABETES
A Holistic Approach

MICHAEL HOFER

How to Manage Diabetes
A Holistic Approach
By Michael Hofer

DISCLAIMER
This book offers nutrition, health, and fitness tips but is only for non-commercial, informational purposes. As the information is not intended to replace medical advice, do not rely on this information as a substitute for professional medical advice, diagnosis, or treatment. You should always consult with a physician or other healthcare professional if you have any questions or before you change anything in your medical treatment, diet, or workout routine.

CONTENTS

INTRODUCTION

It can sometimes be a challenge to manage diabetes. Finding out what works best for you can be overwhelming, especially at the beginning of the diagnosis of prediabetes or diabetes type 1 or 2. It certainly was for me when I was diagnosed with type 1 diabetes at 11. Many years of trial and error followed before I finally found an approach that was not only good for diabetes but also for my health in general.

If you follow the holistic approach in this book with a low-carb diet, low-intensity workouts, and mindful living, you will be rewarded with a healthy lifestyle for life.

The low-carb diet is a distinctive element of this approach. It's not only a diet you follow for a few weeks or months, but you can live with a low-carb diet for the rest of your life as it allows for balanced, healthy nutrition without any extremes. The same applies to low-intensity workouts. You can take a short walk at any age and feel the positive effects on your general health and blood sugar levels, which is the goal for people with prediabetes or diabetes. What about mindful living? Like with the low-carb diet and low-intensity workouts, there are no age limitations. The benefits are for life. Our bodies react to our state of mind. For example, the body releases sugar when we are nervous because of the fight-or-flight response. Being more present in the moment relaxes the mind and body, positively affecting your blood sugar levels. In short,

Combining medical treatment with this holistic approach results in a healthier, happier, and simpler life with diabetes.

Sounds like a big statement? It is, but I'm convinced of it. Don't just try the diet or the workouts alone. Mindful practices like meditation are also not sufficient by themselves. Combine the low-carb diet with low-intensity exercises, and don't forget mindful living. It's the combination of all three that makes the difference. Give it a try and see for yourself.

Ultimately, everyone needs to find their approach to what works for them. This book is to show you what has worked best for me, and I believe it can also be beneficial for other people. Consider everything as an example that you can adjust to your situation and needs.

The book is organized into two parts: Part I focuses on nutrition and how my holistic approach to managing diabetes works. Part II shows you how tasty a low-carb diet can be.

Part I starts with Chapter 1, which provides a more detailed introduction to the first pillar of my holistic approach to managing diabetes.

In Chapter 2, I'll explain more about how the three elements of a low-carb diet, low-intensity workouts, and mindful living play together.

Afterward, we start going into the basics of nutrition. Chapter 3 explains macros and how I propose to manage them in a low-carb diet.

Chapter 4 goes into more detail about carbohydrates and my approach to a low-carb diet.

Chapter 5 is dedicated to the glycemic index, which is a helpful tool for managing diabetes and blood sugar spikes. Combining the glycemic index with a low-carb diet makes a big difference and avoids big swings in your blood sugar.

Chapter 6 introduces the second pillar of the holistic approach, which is mindful living. I'll explain how the body reacts to stress and adrenaline and how it affects blood sugar levels. It also includes a brief overview of different mindfulness techniques.

Chapter 7 discusses the positive effect of physical activity on the body and blood sugar levels. I'll also focus on why low-intensity workouts are the best approach for people with diabetes.

Part II is all about ideas for delicious low-carb meals, starting in Chapter 8 with tips for low-carb breakfasts.

Chapter 9 continues with low-carb salads.

I love seafood, and Chapter 10 gives you ideas for how to implement it into your low-carb diet.

You'll find everything around meat in Chapter 11.

You don't have to give up sweets! Chapter 12 shows you delicious low-carb dessert ideas.

I'm not a medical doctor, so please talk with your doctor or healthcare professional before changing your diet, workouts, or any other part of your lifestyle. Everyone reacts differently, and your diabetes professional will be able to help you.

If you are interested in the latest news about my approach, visit my website: www.healthy-diabetes.com. I regularly post articles and low-carb recipes; you can also download free guides.

Best,

Michael

June 2023

PART I

HOW A HOLISTIC APPROACH TO MANAGING DIABETES WORKS

CHAPTER 1:

A HOLISTIC APPROACH TO MANAGING DIABETES

Living with diabetes can be challenging and requires constant attention. When you have diabetes, you cannot take a day off from managing your diet and medication. It's a 24/7 job. Sounds difficult? It's true that it can sometimes be overwhelming, which is why we need to address it holistically. Living with diabetes is more than just taking medication or following a strict diet; it's about taking a holistic approach to your overall way of living.

> The holistic approach of this book results in a healthy lifestyle whether you have diabetes or not.

In general, by not only using medications but also considering the combination of mind, body, and soul, a holistic approach can help you achieve a healthier lifestyle and better manage your diabetes.

In this chapter, I'll start to discuss the benefits of a holistic approach to diabetes management, from understanding the fundamentals to combining different elements that can help you achieve a healthy, long, and fulfilling life.

Understanding a Holistic Approach

To truly understand the benefits of a holistic approach to managing diabetes, we first need to understand what it means. When I talk about holistic health, I mean a method that focuses on treating a person as a whole, not just a specific issue or symptom. According to the Merriam-Webster Dictionary, holistic means "relating to or concerned with wholes or with complete systems rather than with the analysis of, treatment of, or dissection into parts."[1] My approach is exactly that. I try to understand the different elements but then approach the "complete system," which combines mind, body, and soul. Specifically, it's the combination of your medical treatment with a low-carb diet, low-intensity workouts, and mindful living. However, I don't just talk about specific symptoms of a particular disease or ailment and its medical treatment; it's much more than that. It includes an individual's physical, mental, emotional, and spiritual aspects, recognizing that they are all interconnected and impact one's overall health.

Sounds esoteric? Well, it's more common sense than being esoteric. We all know that we sometimes have days where we feel better than on other days. Do you sometimes have days in the gym where you feel strong and others where you do the basics and feel exhausted? Is it the result of what you ate that day? Or the effect of a difficult day at the office? In all likelihood, it's probably the outcome of many different, sometimes small things. After all, we are a combination of

---

1   "Holistic." Merriam-Webster.com Dictionary, Merriam-Webster, https://www.merriam-webster.com/dictionary/holistic. Accessed 21 Jun. 2023.

many factors, and that is what I want to address with this holistic approach.

When it comes to diabetes management, taking a holistic approach means not only considering traditional medical treatments such as insulin or other medications but also lifestyle factors like stress management, exercise, and nutrition. I'll discuss them in this book by approaching them as a combination as well as separately. For example, only solving the stress element is like taking just one piece of a puzzle.

The Role of Nutrition

Nutrition plays a crucial role in our holistic diabetes management and in every diet. What you consume affects your blood sugar levels, which can result in health issues and complications associated with diabetes if you cannot control it. By adopting healthy eating habits, you can take a proactive approach to managing diabetes. It includes consuming whole foods, which are high in fiber and low in sugar on the glycemic index. Foods like berries, vegetables, whole grains, lean proteins, and healthy fats are all part of a balanced diet that can help improve your health and regulate blood sugar.

Moreover, good nutrition is, in general, an essential factor for a healthy lifestyle and can help to reduce the risk of heart disease and other complications for people with or without diabetes. This is because a healthy diet allows you to control weight, blood pressure, cholesterol levels, and other medical health metrics.

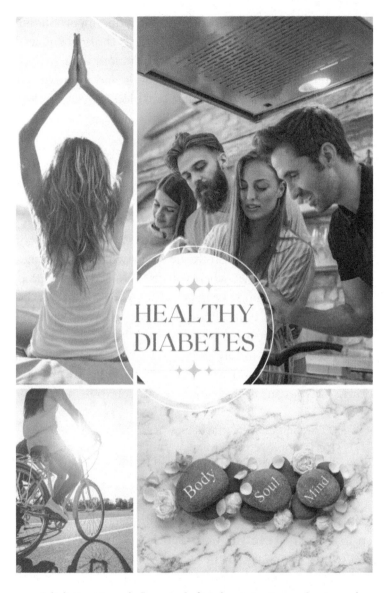

A holistic approach: Low-carb diet, low-intensity workouts, and mindful living

As mentioned, in addition to nutrition, incorporating mind-body techniques for mindful living is also beneficial when managing diabetes. Through meditation, yoga, or similar exercises, we can reduce stress levels and improve our mental health while also helping our blood sugar. So, let's dive in.

Mind-Body Techniques for Mindfulness

Stress is a known trigger for high blood sugar, and high- stress levels can make it harder to manage diabetes. Why is that? Stress releases adrenaline, which again releases the sugar reserves in your body. The reason for this is the fight-or-flight reaction that we need when we are faced with a life-threatening situation. However, when you feel stressed all the time, it means that your body keeps releasing your sugar reserves. The result of this is the high blood sugar levels that need insulin. For many people with diabetes, this means injecting insulin or using an insulin pump. With or without diabetes, this is not healthy, and with diabetes, it results in ups and downs of your sugar levels that are difficult to manage.

> Through mindful practices, you can reduce stress levels, improve your overall health, feel happier, and control your adrenaline and blood sugar.

Also, think about using other approaches for mindful living. While these methods may not be scientifically proven to help, they can still be beneficial. Do whatever allows you to relax and stay in the moment instead of constantly thinking about what happened in the past and may occur in the future. Keep your "monkey mind" under control.[2] The monkey mind never stops thinking; it jumps from thought to thought and doesn't let you relax. Mindfulness techniques

2   Monkey mind is an expression in meditation.

help you calm the monkey mind by focusing more on the current moment.

Some people choose to incorporate acupuncture, yoga, or massage therapy into their mindfulness exercises to help reduce stress, which in turn helps to control your blood sugar. The main goal is to relax from time to time, enjoy the moment, and give your body and mind a break.

Low-Intensity Workouts

In addition to nutrition and mindful living, physical activity is the third component of our holistic approach to managing diabetes. Regular exercise helps everyone, and it's fantastic for people with diabetes. I personally feel the positive effects of workouts for 24–48 hours, which is the reason why my approach is to work out at least every other day. My blood sugar is lower and significantly easier to manage.

Ideally, combine both aerobic and strength training exercises into your workout routine. Walking, biking, or swimming are good examples that improve cardiovascular health and lower blood sugar levels. Working out in the gym can help to build muscle mass and improve bone density. The good news about low-intensity workouts is that you can do whatever you like. You are not limited to specific activities, which results in a more diverse and fun combination of different sports and exercises.

Like with your diet, your exercises need to be tailored to your individual needs and abilities. Talk with your healthcare provider before starting any new exercise programs. It's best to ensure that you are safe to participate.

CHAPTER 2:

UNDERSTANDING MACROS FOR A SUCCESSFUL LOW-CARB DIET

Once you start reading about different diets, you will hear about macros. But what are macros? And how do we use them in our diets? For many, understanding macros is an overwhelming task. In this chapter, I'll provide more information to help you understand them and how they relate to a successful low-carb diet. You'll learn what macros are, how to calculate your daily macro needs, tips to track them successfully, common mistakes to avoid, and the benefits of implementing macros in your low-carb-diet journey. So, let's dive in and take control of your health by creating a macro-friendly meal plan!

What Are Macros and Why Do They Matter?

Let's first discuss what macros are and why they matter. Macros, short for macronutrients, are the three primary nutrients that make up our food: carbohydrates, proteins, and fats. Each macro serves a specific function in our bodies, and the right balance of macros is essential for maintaining good health and achieving our fitness and diet goals.

Carbohydrates provide energy for our bodies and are essential for brain function. Proteins are necessary for building and repairing muscles, as well as other tissues in our bodies. Fats, as well as providing energy, are essential for the absorption of specific vitamins and minerals. Simply put, we need all three macros. However, the amount differs for each group, and different diets use different approaches to distribute the share of the three macros.

Tracking macros can help us get the right balance of nutrients to support our diet goals. By calculating our daily macro needs and tracking our meals, we can make adjustments to meet our goals and keep our bodies healthy and energized.

How to Calculate Your Daily Macro Needs

Tracking our macronutrient intake is fundamental to achieving success with any diet. The recommended daily amount of macros varies depending on a person's needs, goals, and diet. Calculating your daily macro requirements is the first step to ensuring you meet your individual needs.

To calculate this, you'll need to determine your total daily energy expenditure (TDEE), which is the total calories your body burns daily, including activities like working out and everything else. Once you know your TDEE, you can determine your daily macro needs based on your desired ratios of proteins, fats, and carbohydrates. Many websites have calculators to estimate your TDEE. Just Google "total daily energy expenditure (TDEE)," and you will get a helpful list.

A general starting point for a low-carb diet is a macro ratio of 40% protein, 40% fat, and 20% carbohydrates, and I use those ratios in my diet. Like with many things, adjust the percentage based on your preferences and goals. For example, someone who wants to build muscle may wish to incorporate a higher protein ratio, while someone looking to lose weight may want to adjust the carbohydrate and fat ratio.

Tracking your daily macro intake can initially seem overwhelming, but practice makes it easier. A food tracking app can help you keep track of your macros and adjust your nutrition to meet your goals. Let's now look at some other tips for successfully tracking your macros.

Tips for Tracking Macros Successfully

Consistent tracking is crucial for staying on track and meeting your goals. Here are some tips for tracking your macros successfully:

❖ Use a food tracking app: Many apps, such as MyFitness-Pal, can help you track your daily macro intake. Not only will it make tracking easier, but it can also provide valuable insights into your overall nutrition.

❖ Plan ahead: It's essential to plan your meals and prepare your food at home as much as possible. By doing so, you have better control over the macros in your meals, and it'll make tracking easier.

❖ Be consistent: Keeping a log of your meals throughout the day, even on weekends or holidays, can help you stick to your macros better.

❖ Weigh your food: Measuring your food accurately with a food scale is the best way to ensure you consume the right macros.

By following these tips, you can stay on track and progress toward your goals. In the next section, I'll explore some common mistakes to avoid when tracking macros.

Common Mistakes to Avoid

To truly succeed with a low-carb diet, understanding macros is crucial. But even with the best intentions, it's easy to fall into common mistakes that can hinder your progress. One mistake is not accurately tracking your food intake, which can lead to too many carbs or insufficient protein and fat. Additionally, many people overlook the importance of proper hydration while dieting. Dehydration can cause headaches, fatigue, and muscle cramps, derailing any diet plan. Finally, avoid eating too many processed foods marketed as "low carb" but are still high in unhealthy ingredients. By avoiding these common mistakes, you'll be well on your way to achieving success with a low-carb diet.

The Benefits of Understanding Macros for a Successful Low-Carb Diet

By focusing on the ratio of macronutrients in your meals, you can optimize your health, weight loss, and energy levels. But beyond these benefits, understanding macros can also help you become more knowledgeable and aware of the foods you eat. By tracking your macros and learning more about the nutrient content of different foods, you'll make healthier choices and build sustainable habits over time. Ultimately, understanding macros is about more than just achieving short-term weight-loss goals—it's about empowering yourself with the knowledge and skills you need to make informed choices for a healthier, happier life. Remember, patience and dedication are essential to achieving your goals, but with the right mindset and approach, you can take control of your health and reach new heights.

CHAPTER 3:

EVERYTHING YOU NEED TO KNOW ABOUT CARBOHYDRATES

In this chapter, I'm going to focus on carbohydrates. Do you ever feel like carbs are the enemy of good health? That's what you often read in articles and blog posts, but is it true? As mentioned in the chapter before, carbohydrates are essential to our nutrition. They supply energy to our bodies and support our brain function. However, not all carbs are created equal, and choosing the right ones is essential to maintaining a healthy lifestyle. Let's dive into carbohydrates, covering everything you need to know to make informed food decisions. From understanding the different types of carbs to making healthier choices, this chapter has got you covered.

What are Carbohydrates?

Carbohydrates are a macronutrient that provides energy to our bodies. When we eat carbohydrates, the body breaks them down into glucose, which it uses for fuel. The glucose is transported through our bloodstream to provide the necessary energy for our muscles and brain to function. However, the rate at which glucose is absorbed and utilized varies depending on the type of carbohydrate consumed.

Simple carbohydrates, like those found in processed foods, are digested and absorbed quickly, creating a sudden spike in blood sugar levels. These spikes are usually followed by a sudden drop in blood sugar levels, leading to feelings of lethargy and hunger and, in some cases, even mood swings.

On the other hand, complex carbohydrates, which you can find in whole grains, fruits, and vegetables, take longer to digest and are absorbed more slowly. It results in a steady supply of glucose, providing long-lasting energy and preventing blood sugar levels from fluctuating rapidly. You can see how understanding how carbohydrates work in our bodies is crucial for making better choices.

In a low-carb diet, you reserve about 20% of your nutrition for carbohydrates. And this is what I'm proposing in my approach to managing diabetes. Complex carbohydrates are the better choice because they avoid having that up-and-down impact on your blood sugar.

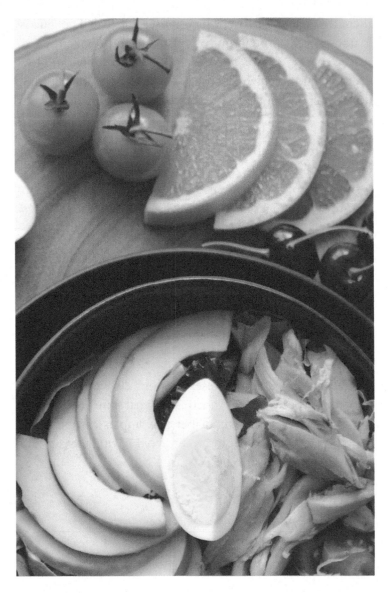

Carbohydrates are an essential element of your nutrition.

CHAPTER 4:

HOW THE GLYCEMIC INDEX CAN HELP MANAGE BLOOD SUGAR

Do you struggle with managing your blood sugar levels? If so, you're not alone. Over 34 million Americans have diabetes, and many more have prediabetes. The glycemic index is one tool that can help you manage your blood sugar. Understanding how different foods affect your blood sugar levels can help you make better choices, thus preventing spikes and crashes. I'll dive into the proven techniques for managing blood sugar with the glycemic index, including choosing the right foods, combining them effectively, and monitoring your progress. Whether you're new to the glycemic index or looking for more tips, this chapter has everything you need to take control of your blood sugar levels and enjoy a healthier life.

Understanding the Glycemic Index

The glycemic index is a ranking system that measures how quickly carbohydrates in food are broken down into glucose and absorbed into the bloodstream. Foods that are high on the glycemic index (GI) are absorbed rapidly and cause a quick increase in blood sugar levels, while those that are low on the GI are absorbed more slowly and result in a gradual rise. Look at the graph below from Harvard Health.

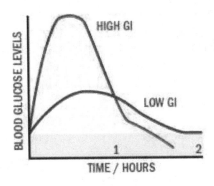

Harvard Health[3]

So, which foods are at what level of the GI? Here are some examples, but go ahead and Google "glycemic index food chart" to get a more comprehensive list.

❖ Low glycemic index (55 or less): Examples are berry fruits and vegetables, beans, minimally processed grains, low-fat dairy foods, and nuts.

3   Harvard Health Publishing. (2023, April 14) "A good guide to good carbs: The glycemic index." Harvard Medical School. https:// www.health.harvard.edu/healthbeat/a-good-guide-to-good-carbs-the-glycemic-index#:~:text=Choose%20low%20glycemic%20foods%20 1%20Low%20glycemic%20index,Cream%20of%20Wheat%20and%20 Mini%20Wheats.%20More%20items

❖ Moderate glycemic index (56 to 69): White and sweet potatoes, corn, brown rice, breakfast cereals without sugar,
and whole grain wheat.

❖ High glycemic index (70 or higher): White bread, rice
cakes, chips, most crackers, bagels, cakes and sweet
treats, doughnuts, croissants, most packaged breakfast
cereals, cookies, potatoes, fries, tropical fruits such as
watermelon and pineapple, and sweetened (with sugar)
dairy products such as fruit yogurts.

By choosing foods low on the GI, you can help prevent
spikes in blood sugar levels and maintain more stable energy
throughout the day. Pairing carbohydrates with protein or
healthy fats can also help slow digestion and prevent blood
sugar spikes—for example, have a piece of whole grain toast
with avocado and a boiled egg for breakfast instead of sug-
ary cereal. Being mindful of the GI and choosing the right
foods can help maintain stable blood sugar levels and improve overall health.

Monitoring Your Progress

You can effectively manage your blood sugar levels by being
mindful of what you eat. The best step-by-step approach to
getting better is to monitor your progress and adjust your
diet regularly based on your learning.

One way to do this is by tracking your daily food intake and
blood sugar readings. It can help you identify patterns and
change your diet and exercise routine. For example, if your
blood sugar levels tend to spike after eating a particular type
of food, you can adjust your diet accordingly.

Another way to monitor your progress is by regularly
checking in with your healthcare provider. They can help you

interpret blood sugar readings and guide your medication or insulin dosage.

In addition, it's essential to be aware of other factors that can impact your blood sugar levels, such as stress and sleep. By keeping track of these factors and how they affect your blood sugar readings, you can change your lifestyle as necessary.

Monitoring your progress is an integral part of managing your blood sugar levels and promoting overall health and well-being. By taking a holistic approach to your health and making adjustments as necessary, you can successfully manage your blood sugar and lead a healthy, fulfilling life.

The Glycemic Index Can Be a Game-Changer

By understanding the GI, choosing the right foods, combining them effectively, and monitoring progress, you can take control of your diabetes and enjoy a more stable life. Remember, managing your blood sugar with the GI is a powerful tool, but it's not the only one. Combining it with other strategies can be even more effective in managing diabetes. So, take action and put these tips into practice today. As you embark on this journey, remember that a journey begins with the first step. By taking that step today, you will be one step closer to enjoying the benefits of better blood sugar control.

CHAPTER 5:

POSITIVE EFFECTS OF MINDFULNESS FOR DIABETES

After examining the details of nutrition and a low-carb diet in the previous chapters, let's discuss the next cornerstone of our holistic approach: mindful living. It's a fundamental element to improve your diabetes management and reduce stress. But first, what is mindfulness?

> Mindfulness is a practice that involves bringing your attention to the present moment, taming your ever-active busy monkey mind, and being in the here and now.

Sounds easy, right? But it isn't. Our minds are conditioned to reconsider what we did and said in the past, and we constantly think about the future and what may happen. It's actually rather difficult for us humans to "just" stay in the moment.

Mindfulness and Diabetes

Constantly jumping from one thought to the next and thinking about what happened in the past and what can happen in the future creates stress. The problem with stress is that it goes hand in hand with adrenaline, which increases blood sugar by stimulating the liver to release glucose into the bloodstream. Adrenaline also reduces the insulin the pancreas releases, which can further increase blood sugar levels. It is crucial in a life-threatening situation because the released sugar helps our muscles act quickly, but—luckily—most of us are not in such dangerous situations daily.

In summary, stress produces adrenaline, which releases sugar from the liver and reduces insulin production in the pancreas. The result is high sugar for people with diabetes and a constantly working pancreas for people without diabetes. It's simply unhealthy.

This is especially true if you regularly feel stressed, as it creates significant health problems over time. It's difficult for people with diabetes because balancing this increased sugar is challenging. I know from experience that it sometimes takes hours to bring blood sugar down to normal levels if adrenaline is the reason for the increase, even by injecting insulin.

How can mindfulness help? As mentioned, mindfulness involves shifting your focus to the present moment and becoming more aware of your thoughts and feelings without judgment. It relaxes the body and mind, and by doing so, you significantly reduce stress, which positively affects your blood sugar levels. This is why it's one of the cornerstones in my approach to managing diabetes: Mindfulness helps minimize blood sugar volatility.

Other Benefits of Mindfulness

One of the most significant benefits of mindfulness is its ability to reduce stress and anxiety. As mentioned before, when we are mindful, we focus on the present moment rather than dwelling on the past or worrying about the future. It helps us to break the cycle of negative thoughts and emotions that can lead to stress and anxiety. Studies have shown that mindfulness can reduce symptoms of anxiety and depression and improve overall well-being.

Not only that, but mindfulness can also improve our quality of sleep. By calming the mind and reducing stress, mindfulness helps us to fall asleep faster and stay asleep longer. In fact, when it comes to treating insomnia, studies have shown that mindfulness can be just as effective as medication.

It can also help us develop emotional resilience, which is the ability to bounce back from difficult situations. By teaching us to be present and non-judgmental, mindfulness helps regulate our emotions and allows us to respond to challenging situations more constructively. This serves us to feel more in control and less overwhelmed by difficult emotions.

It also boosts the immune system. By reducing stress, mindfulness can help us fight infections and illnesses more effectively. Studies have also shown that mindfulness can increase the production of antibodies, which are essential for fighting off disease.

Mindfulness can improve cognitive function, including attention, memory, and decision-making. By training the brain to focus on the present moment, mindfulness can improve our concentration and focus on tasks. This can be especially helpful for those with ADHD or other attention-related disorders.

Mindfulness Techniques

After learning that being mindful has many positive effects, including with your diabetes, the big question is how to get there. What techniques can you use to get to a state of being present?

You probably think of yoga and meditation when you think of mindfulness; however, you can use whatever works for you. There are many ways to achieve it, and everybody is different when choosing the right approach. Let's now discuss a few of the more common techniques.

Mindful Breathing and Meditation

Simply taking a few minutes out of your day to focus on your breath can significantly impact your diabetes management. Mindful breathing and meditation can help reduce stress and bring a sense of calm to your mind and body. To get started, find a quiet space where you can sit comfortably and set aside distractions. Begin by taking a few deep breaths, inhaling through your nose, and exhaling through your mouth. Focus your attention on the sensation of the breath moving in and out of your body. If your mind starts to wander, gently redirect your attention back to your breath. Try practicing mindful breathing and meditation for just a few minutes daily and observe the benefits it can bring to your diabetes management routine. This technique can also help you transition into other mindfulness practices, such as body scans and sensory awareness.

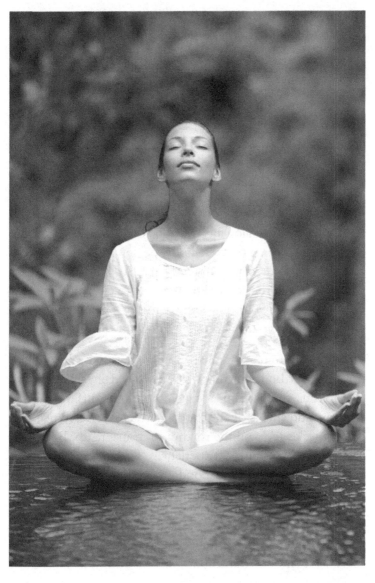

Meditation to relax the body and mind has positive effects on diabetes.

Body Scans and Sensory Awareness

In addition to mindful breathing and meditation, body scans and sensory awareness can be helpful techniques for managing diabetes. These practices involve focusing on different parts of your body and becoming aware of the physical sensations you are experiencing. By doing so, you can increase your overall body awareness and learn to better respond to your body's needs.

To start a body scan, find a quiet and comfortable place to sit or lie down. Begin by closing your eyes and taking a few deep breaths, allowing your body to relax. Then, slowly focus on each part of your body, beginning with your toes and working your way up to your head. As you focus on each part, notice any sensations you feel, such as warmth, tingling, or tension. Take your time and try to stay present in the moment, allowing your mind to let go of any distractions.

Sensory awareness involves paying attention to the sensations in your body as you go about your daily activities. For example, as you eat a meal, take note of the different tastes, textures, and smells of the food. As you exercise, notice how your muscles feel and the rhythm of your breath. By staying aware of these sensory experiences, you can better understand how your body responds to stimuli and adjust your diabetes management routine accordingly.

Body scans and sensory awareness are fantastic techniques to incorporate into your mindfulness practice. They can also serve as a smooth transition into practicing mindful eating and exercise, which we will explore next.

Mindful Eating and Exercise

Mindful eating and exercise involve being present in the moment and paying attention to what your body needs. For example, instead of mindlessly snacking or overeating, take note of your hunger and fullness cues. As you exercise, focus on your body and how it feels rather than distracting yourself with music or TV.

By incorporating mindfulness into your eating and exercise habits, you may be able to make healthier choices and manage your diabetes more effectively. Additionally, being mindful while eating and exercising can help you cultivate a deeper appreciation of your body and what it can do.

As mentioned, practicing sensory awareness and body scans can help you transition into mindful eating and exercise. With that in mind, stay attuned to your body's sensations to become more aware of how different foods and activities affect you. This awareness can help you develop a more informed and mindful approach to your diabetes management.

Mindful Moments: How to Make Mindfulness a Part of Your Daily Routine

Let's explore some practical ways to make mindfulness a part of your routine, from starting your day to creating mindful moments throughout the day. Stick with me here, and you'll come away with a toolkit for a more centered and peaceful life.

Start Your Day with Mindfulness

One way to incorporate mindfulness into your daily routine is to start your day with intention. Rather than immediately reaching for your phone or jumping into your to-do list, take a few minutes to sit quietly and focus on your breath. It can ground you and set a positive tone for the rest of your day.

Incorporate Mindfulness into Your Commute

As you continue incorporating mindfulness into your daily routine, consider how to extend this practice to your commute. A mindful commute can help set the tone for the rest of your day, allowing you to arrive at your destination feeling calm and centered. Perhaps you can walk or bike to work instead of driving, allowing you to connect with the present moment and enjoy the scenery around you. If public transportation is your go-to, take a few deep breaths and focus on the present moment instead of getting lost in your thoughts. Being present and mindful during your commute can start your day on the right foot.

Bring Mindfulness to Your Workday

Start by taking a few deep breaths and setting an intention for the day. Consider writing down your priorities and goals, which will help keep you focused and mindful throughout your workday. When you sit down to work, take a moment to assess your body and posture. Adjust your chair or stretch your legs to be comfortable and relaxed.

As you work, be present and mindful of your actions and thoughts. Avoid multitasking and give your full attention to one task at a time. Take breaks throughout the day to stand up, stretch, and move your body, which will help you stay energized and focused.

If you feel stressed or overwhelmed, take a moment to breathe deeply and refocus your thoughts. Consider taking a short walk outside to get fresh air or practicing a quick meditation or mindfulness exercise.

You can stay focused, productive, and centered by bringing mindfulness to your workday. And when you leave work at the end of the day, you can feel satisfied and accomplished knowing that you approached your day with mindfulness and intention.

Make Mindfulness a Part of Your Evening Routine

Continuing your mindfulness practice beyond the workday can help you wind down and decompress while setting you up for a more restful night's sleep. As you prepare for bed, take a few minutes to reflect on the day's events and how you approached them. Did you remain present and focused? Were there moments when you could have been more mindful?

Take note of any improvement areas and plan to prioritize mindfulness the following day. Consider incorporating a brief meditation or breathing exercise into your evening routine to cultivate calm and relaxation further.

By making mindfulness a part of your evening routine, you'll carry the benefits of the practice into your waking and sleeping hours. There are plenty of opportunities throughout the day to create mindful moments and continue building your practice.

Incorporating mindfulness into your daily routine can be a game-changer. By starting your day with mindfulness, integrating it into your commute, workday, and evening routine, as well as creating mindful moments throughout your day, you can experience a more present and focused life. As you begin to make this practice a part of your daily routine, remember to start small and build from there.

The benefits are worth it, especially when you have diabetes. As discussed in this chapter, stress produces adrenaline, which releases blood sugar reserves and makes managing your diabetes significantly more difficult.

So, take a deep breath, tune into the present moment, and join the millions of people who have discovered the powerful impact of mindfulness in their lives.

CHAPTER 6:

LOW-INTENSITY WORKOUTS AND DIABETES

I f you're anything like most people, you likely think that you need to push yourself to the absolute limit to make significant progress at the gym. After all, no pain, no gain, right? But what if there was a more sustainable way to achieve long-term fitness success? Well, I have some good news for you: there is—low-intensity workouts. In this chapter, I'll explain why these workouts are so effective and how they can help you achieve your fitness goals.

Benefits of Low-Intensity Workouts

Let's start with a look at the many benefits of low-intensity workouts.

Low-Intensity Workouts Are Sustainable

One of the most significant benefits of low-intensity workouts is their sustainability. You won't dread going to the gym daily because the activities are not intense enough to leave you feeling drained. It makes it easier to stick to a workout routine, which is critical for long-term fitness success. In addition, low-intensity workouts are less likely to cause injury, so you won't have to take lengthy breaks from exercising. It's a win-win situation.

Low-intensity workouts are also easy to modify, thus making them ideal for people of all fitness levels. You can adjust the exercise based on your current fitness level or any injuries you may have. As you get more comfortable with the activity, you can gradually increase the intensity to keep challenging yourself.

Moreover, you can do them anywhere, anytime, which means you can integrate them into your daily routine. This is especially important if you have a busy schedule and can't commit to going to the gym regularly.

Low-Intensity Workouts Boost Your Metabolism

Low-intensity workouts, such as walking or yoga, have been shown to boost your metabolism. When you engage in low-intensity exercise, your body burns calories, even if it's not as much as when doing high-intensity exercise. This is because low-intensity training is typically done longer, such as a 30-minute walk, which can burn more calories than a 10-minute sprint.

Moreover, low-intensity workouts can also help increase your muscle mass, further boosting your metabolism. Building muscle is important because it requires more energy to maintain than fat. This means that the more muscle you have, the more calories your body burns at rest.

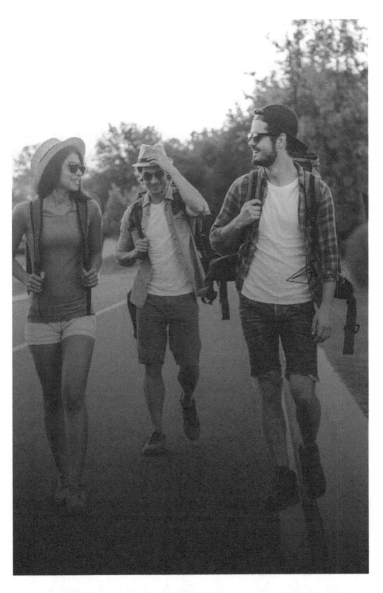

Low-intensity workouts like hiking are perfect for diabetes.

Incorporating low-intensity exercise into your daily routine can help your body burn more calories and become more efficient at burning fat. Plus, it's a great way to get moving and keep your body healthy without putting too much stress on your joints.

Low-intensity workouts can also help reduce stress, which we already know is essential to overall health and fitness. Let's explore this further in the next section.

Low-intensity workouts can be the secret to long-term fitness success for good reasons. Not only do they burn more calories and help your body become more efficient at burning fat, but they also reduce stress. The latter is crucial because stress can lead to many health problems, including weight gain and decreased immunity. So, how exactly do low-intensity workouts help reduce stress?

When you engage in low-intensity exercise, your body releases endorphins which are natural mood boosters. These feel-good chemicals can help you feel more relaxed and calmer, counteracting the adverse effects of stress. Additionally, exercise programs, such as yoga or Pilates, often include mindful breathing techniques that can further reduce stress levels. The slow, deliberate movements of these workouts and the focus on the breath can help quiet your mind and lower stress hormone levels.

Reducing stress through low-intensity exercise not only offers immediate benefits but can also lead to long-term health benefits. When stress levels are high, your body produces high cortisol levels—a hormone that can lead to weight gain and chronic health problems. Incorporating low-intensity workouts into your routine can lower cortisol levels and protect your health in the long run.

Moreover, low-intensity exercise can be a great way to switch up your routine and beat workout boredom.

Low-Intensity Workouts Allow for More Variety

In addition to the health benefits, low-intensity workouts also allow for more variety in your fitness routine: exercises like yoga, hiking, and swimming can help you switch up your routine and keep your activities interesting. Trying new low-intensity exercises can also challenge your body in different ways and provide a break from the high-intensity, high-impact activities that can ultimately lead to burnout or injury.

For example, incorporating low-intensity workouts like Pilates or barre into your practice can help improve your balance, flexibility, and core strength. While mixing in other low-intensity exercises like brisk walking or leisurely bike riding can give your joints a break from the pounding they may experience during high-intensity workouts like running or CrossFit. You can also avoid boredom and burnout while reaping the health benefits of regular physical activity. And as I'll discuss in the next section, low-intensity workouts can also help build endurance and improve overall fitness levels.

Low-Intensity Workouts Can Build Endurance

By incorporating a variety of low-intensity workouts into your fitness routine, you can reap the benefits of consistent physical activity without risking burnout or injury, improve flexibility and core strength, improve overall fitness levels, and set yourself up for long-term success. This is because, while being less challenging than high-intensity exercises, they can still be difficult enough to elevate your heart rate and improve your cardiovascular health.

Building endurance through low-intensity workouts can also prepare your body for more challenging activities in the future. As your body becomes more accustomed to regular physical activity, you can tackle more intense workouts with greater ease and endurance. This can be particularly beneficial for those just starting a fitness journey or who may have taken a break from regular physical activity for a while.

Low-Intensity Workouts Can Help You Stay Active for Life

Building endurance can have long-lasting benefits beyond improving your fitness levels. By incorporating low-intensity activities into your routine, you will find that staying active becomes easier and more enjoyable, and you will also set yourself up for a lifetime of staying active. You may even look forward to your next workout, whether a leisurely walk or a gentle yoga class. Additionally, low-intensity exercises are generally low-impact, making them easier on your joints and muscles and less likely to result in injury.

Incorporating low-intensity workouts into your routine can help you establish a healthy and sustainable fitness habit. By making physical activity a regular part of your life, you are more likely to stick with it and reap the long-term benefits. In the next section, I'll explain how low-intensity workouts can be a particularly effective form of exercise for those with diabetes.

~ ❖ ~

Low-intensity Workouts are Great for Diabetes

For people with diabetes, regular exercise is crucial for managing the condition and maintaining overall health. Low-intensity workouts can be an excellent way for individuals with diabetes to get the physical activity they need without putting too much stress on their bodies.

One of the most significant benefits of low-intensity exercise for those with diabetes is improved blood sugar control. Activities like walking and gentle yoga increase insulin sensitivity and help the body to use glucose more effectively. It can lead to lower blood sugar levels and a decreased risk of diabetes-related complications.

In addition to improving blood sugar control, low-intensity workouts can help with weight management and cardiovascular health. Regular exercise can help lower blood pressure and cholesterol levels, reducing the risk of heart disease and stroke.

It's important to note that individuals with diabetes should always consult with their healthcare provider before starting a new exercise routine. They may need to monitor their blood sugar levels more closely during and after exercise and adjust their medication or insulin as needed.

Overall, low-intensity workouts offer a safe and effective way for individuals with diabetes to stay active and manage their condition. So, if you're looking for a sustainable fitness habit that works for you, consider incorporating low-intensity exercise into your routine. Your body (and your mind) will thank you!

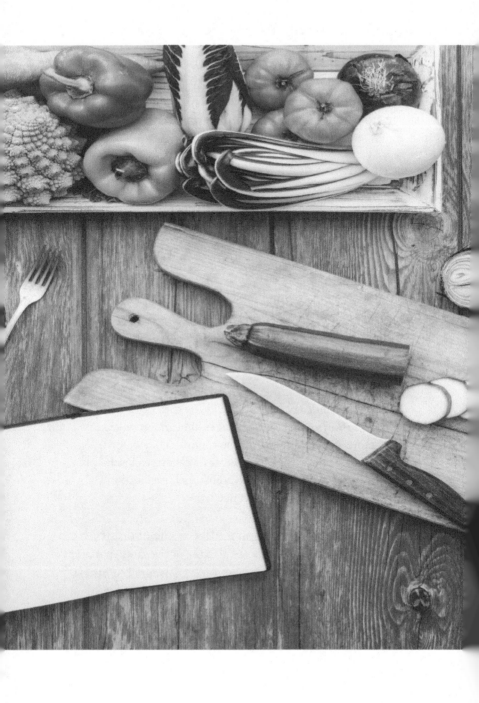

PART II
LOW-CARB RECIPES

CHAPTER 7:

LOW-CARB BREAKFAST ON THE GO

A re you tired of skipping breakfast or settling for carb-heavy options on busy mornings? Finding quick and easy breakfast options can be a struggle if you're following a low-carb lifestyle. But fear not—we've got you covered. In this chapter, I'll share tips and tricks for enjoying a delicious, low-carb breakfast on the go.

Egg Muffin Cups

A great make-ahead option for a low-carb breakfast on the go is an egg muffin cup. These are easy to prepare in advance and can be stored in the fridge or freezer for a quick and convenient breakfast option.

To make egg muffin cups, simply whisk together eggs and your choice of vegetables, cheese, and protein. Pour the mixture into greased muffin cups and bake until set. These can be made in batches and customized to your taste preferences for a satisfying and delicious breakfast.

If you're short on time in the morning, grab a muffin cup on your way out the door for a protein-packed start to your day. Making breakfast ahead of time doesn't have to be complicated, and these egg muffin cups are an excellent option for anyone looking for a convenient and filling low-carb breakfast on the go.

Energizing Smoothies

One of the best things about smoothies is their versatility. You can make them with virtually any combination of fruits and vegetables, which means there's a smoothie recipe out there to suit just about everyone's taste preferences.

To keep your smoothie low carb, be sure to choose low-sugar fruits and vegetables like spinach, kale, berries, and avocado. You can also add in a scoop of protein powder or some Greek yogurt for an extra boost of protein.

Need some inspiration? Here are a few low-carb smoothie recipes to try:

❖ Berry Green Smoothie: Blend together spinach, kale, almond milk, frozen berries, and a scoop of protein powder for a nutrient-packed breakfast on the go.

❖ Chocolate Avocado Smoothie: If you're in the mood for something a little more indulgent, try blending avocado, unsweetened cocoa powder, almond milk, and a touch of stevia for a creamy, chocolatey treat.

❖ Tropical Sunrise Smoothie: Blend together frozen pineapple, mango, banana, and coconut milk for a refreshing and energizing breakfast smoothie.

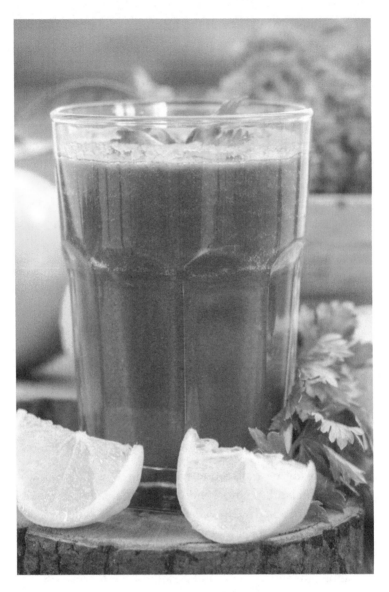

Green smoothie

If smoothies aren't your thing, don't worry. Up next, I'll be sharing our favorite low-carb granola bar recipes.

Low-Carb Granola Bars

Are you looking for a convenient and satisfying breakfast option that won't derail your low-carb diet? Try making your low-carb granola bars at home! Not only are they easy to make, but you can control the ingredients and customize them to your liking.

One recipe to try is a peanut butter and chocolate chip granola bar made with almond flour, shredded coconut, and keto-friendly sweeteners like erythritol or stevia. Another option is a berry and almond granola bar made with a mix of nuts, seeds, and dried fruit like goji berries and cranberries.

Whichever recipe you choose, these granola bars are perfect for busy mornings on the go. Pair them with fruit and nuts for a well-rounded breakfast that keeps you fueled until lunchtime.

Portable Yogurt Parfaits

Another great option for a low-carb breakfast on the go is a portable yogurt parfait. Not only are they easy to make, but they're also a delicious way to start your day. Begin by choosing a low-carb yogurt, preferably unsweetened, and layer it with your favorite berries or chopped nuts.

Assemble the parfait in a portable container, such as a mason jar or a plastic to-go cup with a lid. This will allow you to take your breakfast with you, whether commuting to work or running errands.

Whichever recipe you choose, these granola bars and yogurt parfaits are perfect for busy mornings on the go. Pair them with fruit and nuts for a well-rounded breakfast that keeps you fueled until lunchtime.

CHAPTER 8:

LOW-CARB SALADS YOU'LL LOVE

Are you tired of bland salads that leave you feeling unsatisfied? Do you want to eat healthy without sacrificing flavor? Look no further than the low-carb salad recipes I'll discuss in this chapter. Packed with nutrients and bursting with flavor, these salads will indeed become your go-to for lunch and dinner. From creative greens to protein-packed options and flavorful veggies, I'll explore how you can enjoy a delicious, guilt-free meal. Plus, I'll share some homemade salad dressing recipes to help you take your salads to the next level. Get ready to say goodbye to boring salads and hello to a world of delicious, nutritious options.

Get Creative with Greens

While greens like lettuce, spinach, and kale are often the base for salads, there are many other options to mix things up and add variety to your meals. Try arugula, watercress, or radicchio for a bold and peppery flavor. Add some fresh herbs like mint or cilantro to your greens for a sweeter taste. You can also experiment with different textures by adding shredded cabbage or thinly sliced fennel.

Now that you have some creative ideas for your greens, let's move on to protein-packed options to add more substance to your salads.

Protein-Packed Salad Ideas

Salads can be a great way to pack in some veggies, but they often lack the protein required to keep you full. But fear not—there are plenty of ways to bulk up your salads with protein! One option is adding some grilled chicken or steak, but vegetarian and vegan options are also plentiful. Add some hard-boiled eggs, tofu, chickpeas, or even quinoa to your bowl for a filling and satisfying meal.

But don't stop at just one source of protein—mix it up for even more variety! Top your salad with a mix of nuts and seeds like almonds, sunflower seeds, or hemp hearts for some extra crunch and protein. Or, opt for some crumbled feta cheese or diced avocado, which adds protein and healthy fats.

Adding some protein will make your salad a complete meal that keeps you full and satisfied for hours. And the best part is that there are endless possibilities for flavor combinations, so you'll never get bored.

Now that you've got your protein fix, let's incorporate healthy fats and flavorful veggies for a truly satisfying salad.

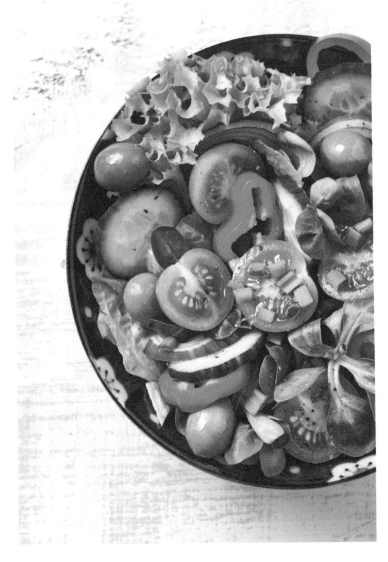

Salads are great for a low-carb diet.

Healthy Fats and Flavorful Veggies

With the addition of protein, your low-carb salad is already a win. But to make it even better, incorporate some healthy fats and flavorful veggies for a truly satisfying meal. Avocado, nuts, seeds, and olive oil are all great sources of healthy fats that add delicious creaminess and crunch to your salad. Don't be afraid to experiment with different veggies, too: roasted Brussels sprouts, sautéed mushrooms, and grilled zucchini are just a few examples of flavor-packed additions that will take your salad to the next level. And the best part? These ingredients are all low in carbs, high in fiber, and loaded with nutrients to energize you.

Dress it Up: Homemade Salad Dressing Recipes

If you want to take your low-carb salad to the next level, consider making your own dressing. It's a healthier option than store-bought varieties, incredibly simple, and allows you to customize the flavors to suit your taste preferences.

One of the easiest homemade dressings to make is a classic vinaigrette. Combine olive oil, vinegar (such as balsamic, red wine, or apple cider), Dijon mustard, and some sweeteners. Whisk everything together and season with salt and pepper to taste. This dressing is perfect with a simple arugula salad or roasted vegetables like Brussels sprouts or asparagus.

If you want something with more tang, try making a creamy avocado dressing. Combine avocado, Greek yogurt, lime juice, garlic, and cilantro in a blender or food processor. Blend until smooth and season with salt and pepper. This dressing is perfect on a salad with grilled chicken or shrimp and pairs well with crunchy fresh veggies like bell peppers or cucumber.

Try making a blue cheese dressing at home for a more indulgent dressing. Combine crumbled blue cheese, sour cream, buttermilk, and garlic for a delicious and tangy dressing. This pairs perfectly with a salad topped with grilled steak or roasted mushrooms.

By making your own salad dressing, you can easily cater to your own tastes and preferences and avoid any unwanted added sugars or preservatives. So next time you're putting together a low-carb salad, take a few extra minutes to whip up a homemade dressing—your taste buds will thank you for it.

Healthy eating can be both delicious and fulfilling, and these low-carb salads are proof of that. By getting creative with greens, adding protein-packed ingredients, incorporating healthy fats and flavorful veggies, and dressing it up with homemade dressings, you can indulge in guilt-free meals that satisfy your cravings. So next time you're in the kitchen, give one of these recipes a try to enjoy a salad that's both nutritious and satisfying.

CHAPTER 9:

TASTY LOW-CARB SEAFOOD MEALS

Are you tired of the same old chicken and beef on your low-carb diet? Why not mix things up with some delicious and healthy seafood? Not only is it a great source of protein, but seafood also provides numerous health benefits. In this chapter, I'll dive into why seafood is a fantastic addition to a low-carb diet, how to choose the right seafood, tips for pairing it with low-carb vegetables and grains, and some mouthwatering recipes to get you started. Get ready to discover the many ways seafood can enhance your low-carb meal plan.

Why Seafood is a Great Addition to a Low-Carb Diet

Seafood is a nutrient-rich food with high-protein content, low-carb count, and virtually no saturated fat. It also boasts a range of essential vitamins and minerals, such as omega-3 fatty acids, zinc, selenium, and iron—all critical for maintaining good health. Adding seafood to your low-carb diet diversifies your meal plan and can help protect you against several illnesses, including heart disease, stroke, depression, and cognitive decline.

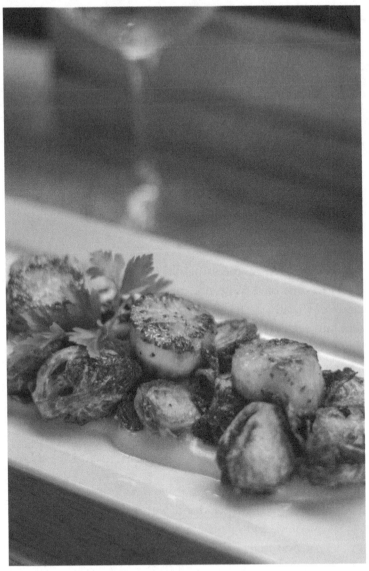

Consider adding seafood to your diet.

However, not all seafood is equal when it comes to carbs. While shrimp, crab, and lobster have no carbs, others, like octopus, mussels, and oysters, contain small amounts. That's why choosing the right seafood is critical when following a low-carb diet. Below is a link to some details from the FDA.[4]

In the next section, I'll share some tips on selecting seafood that is low in carbs and high in nutritional value to maximize the benefits of your diet.

Pairing Seafood with Low-Carb Vegetables and Grains

As I've been discussing, seafood is a fantastic option for those with diabetes, as it's rich in protein and healthy fats. However, to make sure you are getting the most out of your meals, it's important to pair your seafood with low-carb vegetables and grains.

One great pairing is grilled shrimp with roasted asparagus and cauliflower rice. The shrimp provides a good source of protein and healthy fats, while the asparagus and cauliflower rice add fiber and a variety of vitamins and minerals. Another option is to enjoy a salmon fillet with sautéed kale and quinoa. This meal is high in protein, fiber, and healthy fats, making it an excellent choice.

By pairing seafood with low-carb vegetables and grains, you can create well-rounded and nutritious meals that will keep you satisfied and energized. Now that you know how to pair your seafood with low-carb options, let's move on to some delicious recipes.

4   "Nutrition Information for Cooked Seafood (Purchased Raw)." (2018, October 31). FDA: U.S. Food and Drug Administration. https://www.fda.gov/food/food-labeling-nutrition/nutrition-information-cooked-seafood-purchased-raw.

Seafood Ideas for Low-Carb Diets

One great seafood idea is pan-seared scallops with roasted Brussels sprouts. Scallops are a fantastic source of protein and are low in calories, making them an excellent option for those wanting to watch their weight. Meanwhile, the roasted Brussels sprouts add fiber, essential vitamins, and minerals, making this meal healthy and delicious.

Another recipe perfect for low-carb diets is grilled halibut with zucchini noodles. Halibut is full of healthy omega-3 fatty acids while low in calories, thus making it an excellent choice for those looking for a healthy and satisfying meal. The zucchini noodles are a low-carb alternative to regular pasta and add a variety of nutrients and fiber to the dish.

Seafood is not only a delicious addition to any low-carb meal plan, but it also brings many benefits. From its high-protein content to numerous health benefits, it really is a fantastic way to enhance the nutritional value of your meals. By carefully choosing the right seafood and pairing it with low-carb-friendly vegetables and grains, you can create an array of mouthwatering dishes that will leave you feeling satisfied and healthy. So go ahead and try out the seafood recipes in this chapter and explore all the exciting possibilities this fantastic food offers.

CHAPTER 10:

WHY MEAT IS THE PERFECT ADDITION TO YOUR LOW-CARB DIET

Meat has always been a controversial topic regarding health and weight loss. Many quickly eliminate it from their diets in favor of plant-based options or meat substitutes. However, what if I told you that incorporating meat into a low-carb diet could offer numerous benefits for overall health and well-being? In this chapter, I'll dive into why meat is the perfect addition to your low-carb diet. From providing essential nutrients to helping with weight loss and improving gut health, I'll uncover why you should consider adding meat to your meal plan.

Benefits of Meat in Your Nutrition

Let's first look at the many benefits of meat. Meat tastes delicious and offers a plethora of nutrients essential for your body. Apart from being low in carbs and high in protein, it's an excellent source of iron, vitamin B12, and zinc.

Iron is essential for producing red blood cells, while vitamin B12 helps maintain healthy nerve cells and DNA synthesis. Zinc helps in boosting the immune system and maintaining healthy skin. Incorporating meat into your low-carb diet ensures your body gets all the essential nutrients to function effectively.

Meat is Low in Carbs and High in Protein

One of the main reasons why meat is a great addition to a low-carb diet is that it's low in carbs and high in protein. This means you can enjoy meat without worrying about consuming too many carbs, which may spike your blood sugar levels. Instead, you'll get a good dose of protein, which is crucial for building and repairing tissues in your body. Protein is also essential for promoting feelings of satiety, which can help you stay full longer and prevent overeating.

In addition to being low in carbs and high in protein, meat is also a great source of other essential nutrients that your body needs. For example, red meat is rich in iron, which is important for producing red blood cells that carry oxygen throughout your body. Similarly, poultry is an excellent source of vitamin B12, which is vital for maintaining healthy nerve cells and DNA synthesis. Zinc, found in red meat and poultry, is essential for boosting the immune system and maintaining healthy skin.

By incorporating meat into your low-carb diet, you can ensure your body gets all the essential nutrients needed to function effectively. Plus, with its high-protein content and ability to promote feelings of satiety, meat can help you stick to your low-carb diet and achieve your weight-loss goals. Speaking of which, let's take a closer look at how meat can help with weight loss.

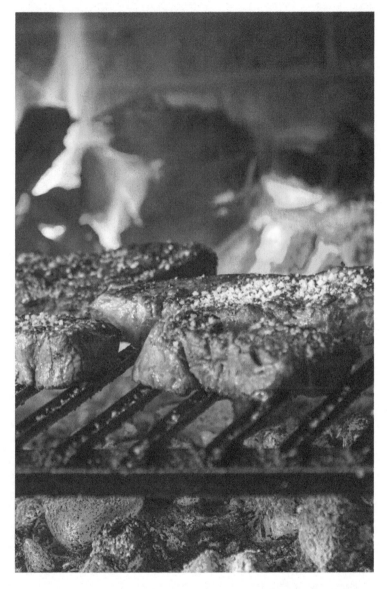

You can use all kinds of meat in your low-carb diet.

Meat Helps with Weight Loss

By incorporating meat into your low-carb diet, you can ensure that your body gets all the essential nutrients it needs, and it helps you achieve your weight-loss goals. Meat has a high-protein content that can promote feelings of satiety, helping you feel fuller for longer periods. This can lead to fewer cravings and less snacking throughout the day, ultimately leading to a calorie deficit and subsequent weight loss.

Studies have also shown that high-protein diets can aid in weight loss and maintenance. Protein has a high thermogenic effect, requiring more energy to digest than carbohydrates or fats. This can increase your metabolism and burn more calories throughout the day.

Meat Improves Gut Health

In addition to its weight-loss benefits, meat consumption can improve gut health. Studies have shown that a diet high in protein can lead to a healthier gut microbiome. This is because the gut microbiome feeds off the protein in your diet, helping to maintain healthy levels of beneficial bacteria.

Moreover, meat is a great source of zinc, which strengthens the gut barrier and can help prevent toxins and harmful bacteria from entering the bloodstream, reducing inflammation and improving overall health.

Meat's ability to provide satiety and reduce cravings also makes it a great addition to any low-carb diet. Let's take a closer look at this in the next section.

Meat Provides Satiety and Reduces Cravings

Incorporating meat into your low-carb diet can help you feel more satisfied and less likely to snack on high-carb, low-nutrient foods. Additionally, studies have shown that consuming protein-rich meals can reduce cravings and decrease the desire to eat late at night.

While it's important to find a balance with your protein intake, adding moderate portions of meat to your low-carb diet can provide you with the necessary protein and satiety to help you reach your health goals. The key is to choose lean cuts of meat and pair them with plenty of non-starchy vegetables for a well-rounded meal.

In addition to weight management benefits, meat consumption has also been linked to improved mood and cognitive function. Meat is a source of essential amino acids needed to synthesize neurotransmitters in the brain. These neurotransmitters regulate mood, memory, and overall cognitive function.

Incorporating Meat in Your Diet

Next, let's explore how to incorporate meat into a healthy and sustainable diet. It's important to choose high-quality meat that is raised sustainably and ethically. Look for grass-fed beef, pasture-raised chicken, and wild-caught fish. These options are better for the environment and animal welfare and are healthier for humans as they contain more beneficial nutrients such as omega-3 fatty acids.

Additionally, balancing meat consumption with various vegetables, fruits, whole grains, and legumes is vital. This not only adds more fiber and nutrients to your diet, but it also helps to reduce the environmental impact of meat consumption. By incorporating plant-based meals into your diet, you can help to reduce greenhouse gas emissions, preserve water resources, and protect biodiversity.

When it comes to meat and sustainability, less is often more. Aim for smaller portions of high-quality meat and incorporate meatless meals into your diet. By making conscious choices about where your meat comes from and how much you consume, you can enjoy the health benefits of meat while also doing your part to protect the planet.

Adding meat to your low-carb diet can provide more than a tasty meal. It offers essential nutrients, low carbs, high protein, and various health benefits, including weight loss, improved gut health, and reduced cravings. You can enjoy a healthy and sustainable diet by choosing organic and grass-fed varieties and pairing them with a variety of vegetables.

CHAPTER 11:

GUILT-FREE LOW-CARB DESSERTS

Do you ever crave something sweet but hesitate to indulge because you're on a low-carb diet? You're not alone. Many struggle to satisfy their sweet tooth while sticking to their health goals. But what if I told you that you can enjoy guilt-free desserts that won't wreck your low-carb diet? Yes, you read that right! In this chapter, I'll provide some mouthwatering low-carb dessert ideas you can indulge in without feeling guilty. It's all covered from chocolatey delights to fruity treats, creamy desserts, baked goodies, and even frozen delicacies!

Chocolatey Delights

One option is chocolate avocado mousse, which swaps heavy cream for avocado to create a creamy and rich dessert. Another favorite is chocolate chia pudding, which combines chia seeds, cocoa powder, and almond milk for a decadent and filling treat. And if you're a fan of dark chocolate, try making some sugar-free chocolate truffles with cocoa powder, coconut oil, and a low-carb sweetener. These treats are just a few examples of how you can indulge your chocolate cravings without breaking your low-carb diet.

Fruity Treats

If you're looking for a refreshing and fruity treat on your low-carb diet, there are plenty of options to satisfy your sweet tooth without the guilt. One popular choice is a berry parfait, which layers fresh berries with whipped cream and a sprinkle of nuts for a light and flavorful dessert. Another option is a small piece of grilled fruit, which brings out the natural sweetness and pairs well with a dollop of Greek yogurt. Try making a low-carb berry cheesecake with a nut crust and creamy filling for a more indulgent option. These fruity treats are a great way to mix up your dessert options and keep your low-carb diet interesting. And if you're craving something more decadent, don't worry—I've got plenty of creamy desserts to indulge in next.

Creamy Desserts

One classic choice is a sugar-free chocolate mousse made with heavy cream, cocoa powder, and a sugar substitute. It's velvety and smooth; you won't miss the sugar. Another way to indulge is with homemade low-carb ice cream made using ingredients like almond milk, heavy cream, and fresh fruit. You can even add in some chocolate chips or nuts for extra texture. Finally, try a low-carb panna cotta made with coconut milk, gelatin, and vanilla extract for a decadent and sophisticated dessert. It's creamy, silky, and the perfect way to end a meal.

Baked Goodies

If you want something warm and comforting, check out these baked goodies for even more low-carb dessert inspiration. A great option is low-carb brownies made with almond flour, cocoa powder, and sugar-free sweeteners. These brownies are indulgent and fudgy, and I promise that you won't even miss the high-carb version. Another classic choice is cheesecake, which can be made low carb by using almond flour or coconut flour for the crust and a sugar substitute for the filling. For a seasonal twist, try making pumpkin pie with a low-carb crust using almond flour and coconut oil. It's a delicious way to enjoy a fall favorite without the carb overload. Now, onto frozen delicacies.

Frozen Delicacies

If you're looking for a dessert option that's both refreshing and low carb, look no further than frozen treats. One tasty option is homemade fruit sorbet, which can be made by blending frozen fruit with sugar-free sweeteners and a splash of lemon juice. This dessert is low in carbs and loaded with vitamins and antioxidants. With these frozen delicacies, you can satisfy your sweet tooth and stick to your low-carb diet at the same time.

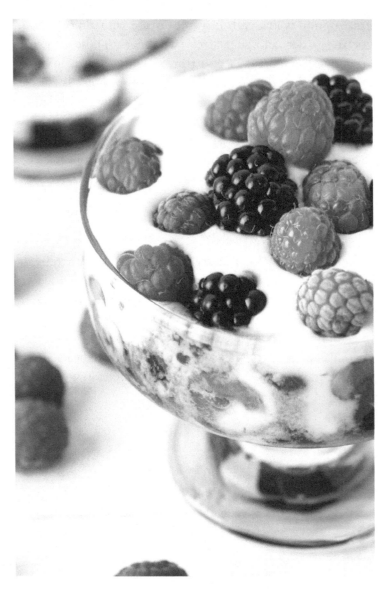

Yogurt with berries for a guilt-free dessert

To wrap this up, sticking to a low-carb diet doesn't have to mean giving up on dessert altogether, far from it, in fact.

You can still indulge in your sweet tooth without feeling guilty, thanks to the guilt-free low-carb desserts in this chapter. From chocolate delights to fruity and creamy desserts to baked goodies, there is something for everyone. They are also great low-carb desserts for people with diabetes. So, what are you waiting for? Give these recipes a try to enjoy a tasty treat without sabotaging your diet. Remember, satisfying your cravings can be healthy too!

CONCLUSION

A life with diabetes can be challenging, but a holistic approach can help you to live a more balanced life with better blood sugar levels. Combining a low-carb diet with low-intensity workouts and mindful living helps achieve a long, healthy, and fulfilling life with diabetes.

But it goes beyond diabetes management; following the outlined principles of a holistic approach is also healthy for people without diabetes. Moreover, you can use it for the rest of your life. A low-carb diet is not only a short-term solution for weight loss like many other diets; it's a healthy, sustainable route to nutrition. The recipes in this book include tasty ideas while demonstrating how diverse a low-carb diet can be.

In a world where more and more people have difficulties dealing with the constant increase in speed and pressure in their professional and personal lives, mindful living is an important factor in balancing outside pressure and our monkey minds. It has been a popular practice for hundreds of years in some areas of the world and is still a great solution to quiet the mind, which has many positive effects on your body. For people with diabetes, it helps to manage the volatility of the blood sugar and the challenging situation of being diabetic.

It's probably not a surprise that sports and working out are beneficial for your body, but the idea of a low-intensity workout may have been new to you. Because you can use whatever exercise you enjoy, there are fewer hurdles to integrating physical activity into your routine. It's also sustainable for the rest of your life, as you can adjust your exercises to your age and fitness level.

One piece of advice that I mentioned a few times in the book is to make it your own. Adjust the diet, mindfulness techniques, and workouts to what fits best with your situation, and always discuss any changes with your healthcare professional. After all, they are there to help you.

Taking "massive action" is a recommendation from Tony Robbins, and it certainly fits this holistic approach. Instead of waiting until next year, start implementing these changes right away. It's never too late.

I hope that you enjoyed the book!

Best,

Michael

About The Author

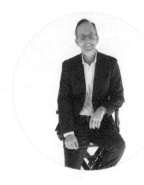

Michael Hofer has been diabetic since his 11th birthday and has developed over the years an approach to achieve a long, healthy, and fulfilling life with diabetes. He has a Ph.D., MBA, MSA, CPA, and went to Wharton for his executive education. He speaks five languages and has a successful management career at an executive level in international companies. Living a healthy, active, and mindful lifestyle is at the center of his personal life and his approach to managing diabetes.

Read more about him and his approach on his website, where you can also download guides and get regular updates. www.healthy-diabetes.com

Made in the USA
Las Vegas, NV
13 September 2023

77509139R00044